INDIGESTION

HEARTBURN
ULCERS
COLITIS
GALL STONES
DIVERTICULITIS
CONSTIPATION
HIATAL HERNIA
PARASITES
HEMORRHOIDS

©1993

Kurt W. Donsbach, D.C., N.D., Ph.D.

Important Notice:
The contents of this book are the opinions and research data collected by the author. It does not purport to give advice on disease treatment or to advise any reader on the proper treatment of any disease. This book is intended for informational purposes only and the author and/or publisher accept no responsibility for any actions of a reader. It is highly recommended that if you have a disease condition, you consult with your physician or healer for professional advice.

©1993   Printed in U.S.A.

Published by: The Rockland Corporation
Tulsa, Oklahoma
800-421-7310

TABLE OF CONTENTS

Table of Contents (cont.)

The Gastrointestinal Tract

It seems that of all the organs we have in the body, the gastrointestinal tract gives us the most frequent problems. If you will take a look at the various areas of this lifeline to your body, it should be obvious that there are many areas that can and do give mankind problems.

It is the purpose of this booklet to give you a different perspective from that of modern medicine for the problems that seem to arise all too often in the 30 plus feet of food processing tube within us. This is not to say that "their" approach is all wrong, it only signifies that I look at such problems in a different way and try to correct them using a more natural approach.

Perhaps we should discuss this for just a moment. Let's look at simple indigestion. The cause of this discomfort is *not* a deficiency of an antacid or other function-aborting chemical. The cause usually revolves around two distinctive situations:

1. A simple case of overeating, stressing the ability of the digestive mechanism beyond the accommodation point. This results in distention, pressure and a feeling of fullness. Normally this will pass in a matter of one or two hours as the digestive ability "catches up." This is a simple circumstance and should not be treated except with peppermint and/or ginger, two herbs that have astounding ability to relieve simple indigestion.

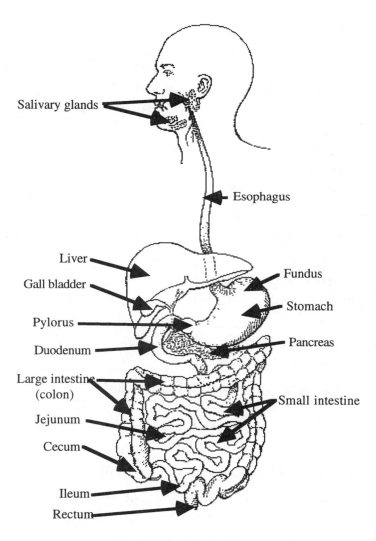

Salivary glands

Esophagus

Liver

Gall bladder

Pylorus

Duodenum

Large intestine (colon)

Jejunum

Cecum

Ileum

Rectum

Fundus

Stomach

Pancreas

Small intestine

The Digestive system

2. The second form of indigestion has the same symptoms but a different cause. The discomfort comes after every meal, regardless how small. Rare exceptions would be meals that are composed primarily of refined carbohydrates which do not remain in the stomach for any of their digestion. The cause of this form is a lack of adequate hydrochloric acid which stimulates the production of the digestive enzyme pepsin in the stomach. This lack can be produced by an inadequate diet which does not furnish the raw materials to make this important acid on demand or an inadequate amount of raw materials to make the enzyme pepsin. There is also a natural slowing down of the production of hydrochloric acid after the age of forty years. Either deficiency can be repaired first with a digestive acid containing the two ingredients and secondly with a recognition of dietary deficiency and the correction thereof.

Modern Medicine Approach

Modern medicine almost always approaches indigestion by recommending a substance which *inhibits* hydrochloric acid – an antacid of some kind. Yes, that approach does relieve the symptoms of discomfort, but it may do so at the expense of far more serious problems. Let me explain.

When you have a stomach full of food that is waiting to be digested but because of a lack of the proper body chemicals to do so you have discomfort. If your response to this discomfort is to add a substance which will further inhibit the ingredients necessary to digest the food, your stomach is faced with a dilemma: what to do with this partially digested mass of food when you have just neutralized an already deficient amount of digestive chemicals with antacids.

The answer is usually a relaxation of the pyloric sphincter (door) at the end of the stomach, allowing the food (even though not completely digested) to leave the area because the possibility of eventual complete digestion is very dim.

This emptying of the stomach contents results in two distinct effects:

1. The exchange of upper intestinal gas and discomfort for lower intestinal discomfort and gas which often is not as socially acceptable.

2. The presence of undigested proteins in the small intestine where they might be absorbed and create allergies. Most allergies come from incompletely digested proteins which have entered the blood stream in some way and cause an overwhelming antibody reaction which may become so sensitive that anytime you consume that food in the future you will have an allergic reaction. Although this scene presumes that there is an inadequate protection against such undigested proteins slipping into the blood stream, many physicians are seriously concerned about a "leaky

gut" syndrome in many of their patients. (more on that later)

By comparing the two approaches which I have just outlined, you can easily see the difference in approach – one is trying to make the symptoms go away, the other looks for the cause and attempts to make the cause go away. Although this may seem as if it is a simplified explanation, it does serve to demonstrate the basic difference in how the wholistic or natural minded healer will look at a problem compared to the modern medicine man who relies almost exclusively on a **medicine to make you well when you are sick that would make you sick if you took it when you were well.**

This difference in philosophy and approach has created a very vicious war with accusations of "quackery" and persecution of those who do not practice according to the "standards of modern medicine." As to what divine right modern medicine has to claim "truth" is far from clear – particularly when one looks at their abysmal record of defeat in the face of chronic degenerative disease which grows year by year in spite of their best research and efforts.

So as you read these pages, you will be exposed to "the other side of the story" when it comes to healing but using the same scientific anatomy and physiology to understand the disease process.

How The Digestive Tract Works

The mere presence or contact of food with the mouth sends a message to the brain which instantly orders the **parotid and salivary glands** to secrete **saliva**, a mixture of water, mucus and a starch digesting enzyme. Sometimes this same reaction can come just from the thought of food or the aroma of food cooking.

The **teeth** grind food into smaller particles and allow better mixing with the saliva. The **tongue** acts to give us a sensation of taste and also acts as a muscular tool to project food into the back of the mouth and into the **throat**. The **epiglottis** acts to cover the windpipe so food does not enter the respiratory tract as it passes backwards and downwards.

The throat connects the mouth to the **esophagus** which is the muscular pipe to the **stomach**. Although gravity usually is of some assistance in getting the food from the throat to the stomach, you can swallow food standing on your head and it will end up in the stomach. This is because of **peristalsis**, a wave-like muscular action which promotes the contents of the esophagus toward the stomach.

The stomach has already been producing **hydrochloric acid** from the moment food entered the mouth. This hydrochloric acid purifies the food content and stimulates the conversion of the enzyme **pepsin** from an inactive form called **pepsinogen**.

Pepsin begins the breakdown of crude food proteins into **polypeptides**, the intermediate stage between proteins and **amino acids**. Although only amino acids can be absorbed through the intestinal tract, the stomach provides a valuable service in beginning the breakdown process. The only food absorbed directly into the bloodstream from the stomach is **alcohol**, all others are absorbed in the small intestine. This also explains the rapidity with which alcohol has an effect on the body.

Once the food has been properly acidified and partially digested, the **pyloric valve** at the end of the stomach opens and allows the **chyme** (the thick juice food has become) to pass into the **duodenum**. The duodenum is almost like a second stomach, here enzymes from the pancreas and bile from the gall bladder are mixed with the chyme and further digestion takes place.

The pancreatic enzymes complete protein and carbohydrate digestion down into amino acids and **glucose** while the bile provides an **emulsifier** which breaks large fat particles down so that the pancreatic enzyme **lipase** can break fats down into **fatty acids** and **glycerol** which can then be absorbed.

Passing from the duodenum to the **small intestine**, the food now goes on a kind of roller coaster ride for about six hours through some twenty feet of small intestine. It comes in contact with billions of **villi**, each of which has several million **microvilli** which further increase the surface area.

The purpose of the villi is to extract the digested nutrients from the chyme as it passes by. In certain diseases these villi are stunted and nonfunctional resulting in extreme malnutrition. (Crohn's Disease is an example.)

Next the food passes into the **large intestine (colon)** where considerable water and some more nutrients are extracted and absorbed.

The colon is only about three feet in length but is at least twice as large in size with its three inch diameter. The remnants of digestion will normally remain here for about **ten hours** before being evacuated. However, in cases of **megacolon** where the colon has stretched out of shape into diameters up to 9 inches, or where there is insufficient **fiber** in the diet to create bulk in the colon, residue may remain there for days before evacuation.

Colonies of so-called "friendly" bacteria attack the residue in the colon and further break it down as well as act as a control for the candida organisms which are present as scavengers in the tract.

And so our journey is complete from intake to excretion along a thirty foot long pathway lined with some of the busiest cells in our body.

INDIGESTION

This term is often misunderstood and misapplied. It should be interpreted as a rather benign, albeit uncomfortable, temporary inability to do a job in the normal amount of time allotted. As we have indicated before, there are basically two reasons for indigestion:

1. Eating too much food.
2. Inadequate supply of hydrochloric acid and/or pepsin.

But we need to examine the problem just a little more closely. Remember that not all foods need to remain in the stomach for extended lengths of time. As an example:

1. Fruit and fruit juices pass through the stomach very quickly if consumed alone.

2. Vegetables in general are not required to stay in the stomach for any length of time if consumed alone. But if high protein vegetables like soy beans or any kind of beans are consumed, they will stay in the stomach for up to three hours.

3. Meats, dairy products, fish and fowl are all destined to stay in the stomach for at least three hours. Although fats do not need to stay in the stomach they are almost always combined with proteins so they are trapped until the protein is digested partially.

Now for the real cause of most **chronic** indigestion. This usually occurs with the person well over forty years of age who has a diminished flow of hydrochloric acid. These individuals soon find out that heavy protein meals cause real distress so they begin to choose more complex carbohydrate meals such as rice, pasta and casserole type dishes.

But they still have their lifelong likes and dislikes as it pertains to foods. So they are constantly putting food combinations into the stomach that are a sure formula for distress. A combination guaranteed to cause problems would be:

> one tall glass of orange juice
> two eggs
> one portion refried beans
> toast or any kind of bread

There is nothing inherently wrong with any of these foods. They are all good foods -- but if you do not have enough hydrochloric acid to sterilize the bacteria in the eggs and beans you will have the bacteria creating fermentation as they contact the sugars in the orange juice. The resulting gas will begin to "blow" up the stomach and give a bloated feeling. The next sensation will be that of burning eructation when the pressure in the stomach so overwhelms the valve at the end of the esophagus that a small amount of the stomach contents are allowed to wash up into the esophagus.

The esophagus does not have the heavy mucous protection of the stomach so the acid will give a sensation of burning and you will likely "taste" the beans. Your immediate reaction is that you cannot eat beans anymore since they are the food causing the problem.

That is not true, but it will make sense at the time. The real problem is an inadequate source of hydrochloric acid which creates fermentation when concentrated proteins (eggs, beans, meat, etc.) are combined at the same time with a high carbohydrate food (fruits, fruit juices, ice cream, etc.). This is the perfect recipe for indigestion.

If you wish to solve the problem, you can use a digestive enzyme combination with each meal you eat and have relative comfort without watching your food combinations. An enzyme combination that will work should contain the following ingredients:

1. hydrochloric acid
2. pepsin
3. pancreatin
4. bile salts
5. optional ingredients:
   papain
   bromelain

In order to ascertain the amount of the above you need, it is best to begin with four or five tablets with each meal and determine comfort level. If four gives you comfort, try three. If that is still fine, try two with each meal. In this way you can find the exact dosage necessary for you better than anyone can prescribe it.

If you do not want to take digestive enzymes on a regular basis you must

FOLLOW THE RULE

The rule is:

Do not combine a concentrated protein with a concentrated carbohydrate at the same meal. Eat small amounts more frequently.

Following this advice will give you comfort instead of discomfort, ease instead of dis-ease.

Acute Indigestion

Acute indigestion occurs when there has been an overloading of the stomach with too much food and drink. And that brings up a common question: ***Should I drink liquids with meals?***

The answer is neither yes or no. Some liquids such as coffee actually stimulate the production of hydrochloric acid and thus help digestion. (I can hear the triumphant cheers now from all you coffee lovers.) A small amount of liquid may also make some rather dry food-stuff mix more readily with the digestive juices in the stomach. The correct answer to the question is moderation in liquid consumption with a meal is perfectly acceptable.

Europeans and early Americans had home remedies for acute indigestion. Two of the favorites were herbs – **peppermint** and **ginger**. These two herbs were commonly drunk as a tea with large feasts to prevent the indigestion which they knew was coming.

Peppermint

What is it about peppermint that could help prevent indigestion? Peppermint is a **carminative** – that is it helps to expel gas. Since most of the problems that are involved in acute indigestion are caused by gas, the use of peppermint is a very good idea. One should be aware that there are two kinds of peppermint – one is the herb, ground and powdered, and the other is peppermint oil. Both have very excellent gastrointestinal properties, but the one you want for upper intestinal gas is the powdered herb or an alcohol extract of the herb known as a tincture. The oil is used for lower intestinal problems and must be specially prepared.

Ginger

Common ginger has a very long history of use in the treatment of a wide variety of intestinal ailments. The Japanese use it extensively as well as many other Eastern cultures. A clue to ginger's usefulness in alleviating gastrointestinal distress was offered in a recent double-blind study, which showed that ginger is very effective in preventing motion sickness. In fact, in this study ginger was shown to be far superior to Dramamine, a commonly used over-the-counter and prescription drug for motion sickness.

Although we are not sure as to the extract action of ginger, it is classified as a carminative and thus makes sense in acute indigestion.

Charcoal

While we are on the subject of natural remedies that are beneficial for acute indigestion, we must discuss charcoal, a time honored remedy which absorbs, or draws to itself, both toxins and gas in the intestinal tract. The historical use of burnt toast as a gastrointestinal remedy is based upon sound reasoning and chemistry.

Simethicone

A surfactant is a substance which acts on the surface of substances it comes in contact with. In the case of simethicone, its action is to cause tiny gas bubbles to join together and create larger bubbles which are easier to eliminate from the body.

Grand Remedy

It would be a grand remedy that contained all four of these effective natural medicines. Imagine carrying a vial of six or twelve capsules containing charcoal, simethicone, ginger and peppermint. Good-bye to acute indigestion!

Heartburn

Essentially heartburn is the same as acute or chronic indigestion in that it results from pressure of an engorged stomach that actually presses on the heart, or it may be caused by the reflux of stomach acids into the esophagus. If these acids are not quickly washed back down into the stomach, they will set up an irritation in the lower esophagus that hurts intensely and in fact may simulate a heart attack. (See diagram below)

It is important not to lie down if you have heartburn and to use something which will relieve gas pressure (The Grand Remedy?) and soothe the esophagus, such as one-third teaspoon of baking soda with a little water.

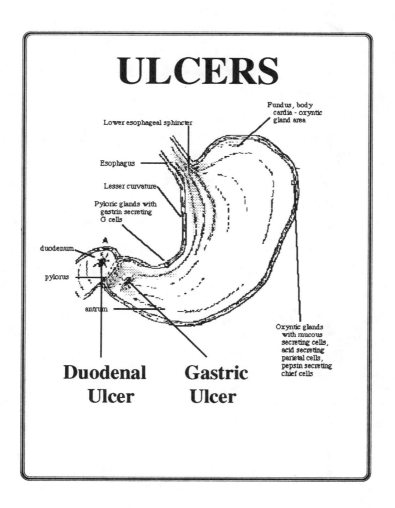

Ulcers

Ulcers are lesions in the stomach or duodenum. Although the commonly held opinion that they are due to an excess secretion of hydrochloric acid is widely accepted, there are several other factors involved.

Looking at the illustration of a cross section of the stomach wall or lining on the next page gives you an idea how deep the mucous lining of the stomach really is. It is only when this lining becomes thinner and less resistant that hydrochloric acid can etch a wound which results in an ulcer. And then only if there is a stimulation to produce extra hydrochloric acid without food in the stomach to soak it up.

An ulcer is almost always preceded by a period of **gastritis**, an inflammation of the stomach mucosa. Symptoms of this condition include a **burning sensation, nausea and sometimes vomiting. Alcohol, smoking and the eating of highly seasoned foods** can bring about an attack and should be avoided until the problem is solved.

Meals should be frequent and without sugar, alcohol or highly seasoned foods. Proteins and fats tend to soothe the membrane while fruits tend to irritate it. Vegetables do not affect gastritis or ulcers negatively so may be consumed without fear.

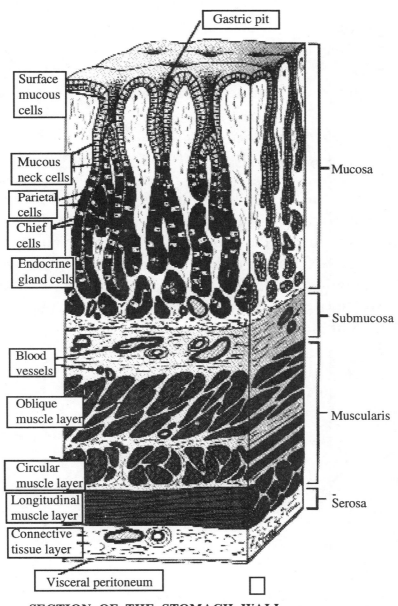

Gastric pit

Surface
mucous
cells

Mucous
neck cells

Parietal
cells

Chief
cells

Endocrine
gland cells

Blood
vessels

Oblique
muscle layer

Circular
muscle layer

Longitudinal
muscle layer

Connective
tissue layer

Visceral peritoneum

Mucosa

Submucosa

Muscularis

Serosa

SECTION OF THE STOMACH WALL

23.

An ulcer located in the stomach is called a gastric ulcer, an ulcer in the duodenum is called a duodenal ulcer. The most common site for ulcers is in the duodenum and the male is overwhelmingly the target of the disease.

80% of duodenal ulcers occur in males
60% of gastric ulcers occur in males

In general, duodenal ulcers occur in the earlier years – from 20 to 30 years of age, and gastric ulcers occur in the later years – from 50 to 60 years of age. Although various remedies are effective in promoting the healing of the ulcer, it is well known that 80% or more of all ulcers will recur within 12 months after therapy is stopped.

Good News – Bismuth

A recent discovery regarding a bacteria called **campo-lacto** (sp) has changed the thinking of most of the informed gastroenterologists who work with ulcer patients every day. The rate of ulcer recurrence after treatment with **bismuth citrate** was less than 10% as compared to the existing treatments which primarily consisted of hydrochloric acid inhibiting substances. The campo-lacto bacteria (sp) evidently is the culprit which disturbs the gastric mucosa to the extent that even normal hydrochloric acid secretion irritates the lining and causes the typical burning ulcer pain.

Extensive research has been accomplished on the use of various bismuth preparations as a method of destroying this bacteria. Hands down, bismuth citrate was the big winner. A preparation on the market uses bismuth but not bismuth citrate – they use **bismuth subsalycilate** which is effective in coating the stomach but not as effective as bismuth citrate in destroying the campo-lacto (sp) bacteria.

This commercial preparation also contains a magnesium/**aluminum** combination which I am opposed to. The EPA limit for aluminum in water supplies is 2 mg per liter (approx. one quart) but an ulcer patient may use several thousand milligrams per day in his constant use of the over-the-counter antacid preparations which are based on the mineral aluminum. This mineral is a common ingredient in food because our soils are so rich in it. Excessive content in the cells has been linked to **Alzheimer's Disease** and other negative conditions of the body.

So my advice is to avoid the high aluminum containing antacids and use a preparation containing bismuth citrate. Such a preparation exists and contains **bismuth citrate, peppermint, ginger, calcium and magnesium**, all in a pleasant tasting liquid form.

This preparation attacks what is now known as the cause of ulcers, and at the same time relieves the symptoms in a totally natural way.

Please Note: Bismuth will turn your stool **dark, even black** and some individuals have panicked upon observing this phenomena because they believe the black color may come from blood in the upper gastrointestinal tract. If you have been taking any form of bismuth and your stool turns dark, relax, it is perfectly normal.

Interesting Research

FIBER 73 — people with recently healed duodenal changed diets. On a random basis, 38 were told to eat lots of whole grain bread, porridge made from wheat, barley or oats, and lots of vegetables, while 35 were told to avoid these foods. After 6 months the following was observed:

Low Fiber Group – 28/35 (80%) in this group had suffered a relapse of ulcers.

High Fiber Group – 17/38 (45%) in this group had suffered a relapse of ulcers.

Rydning A et al. Prophylactic effect of dietary fiber in duodenal ulcer disease. Lancet 2:736-39, 1982.

21 chronic duodenal ulcer patients in a rice-eating area were put on an unrefined wheat diet and 21 continued on their previous rice diet. After 5 years, only 14% of the first group (high fiber diet) had had relapses compared to 81% of the rice (low fiber) diet. A similar 5-year relapse rate (80%) was obtained in a group of 30 patients from another area with a more varied rice diet. This difference may be due to the increased mastication required by the unrefined wheat diet, which is associated with an increase in saliva, lower stomach acidity and reduced bile output. *Malhotra SL. A comparison of unrefined wheat and rice diets in the management of duodenal ulcer. Postgrad Med. J. 54:6-9, 1978.*

VITAMIN A — 52 patients who had had severe physiologic stresses (burns, organ injuries or postoperative organ disturbances) were randomly divided into treatment and control groups. Treatment consisted of water soluble **vitamin A 100,000 IU twice daily (200,000 IU daily)** for adults and 1/2 the dose for children. Additional vitamin A was given if serum vitamin A did not promptly normalize. 63% of the controls but only 18% of the treatment group showed evidence of stress ulcer, a significant difference. Since in burn patients, serum vitamin A often falls from initially normal levels and returns to normal after patients receive a high protein diet, the authors speculate that lack of retinol binding protein is responsible for the drop in vitamin A levels. *Chernow MS et al. Stress ulcer: a preventable disease. J Trauma 12:831, 1972.*

Sixteen patients with chronic gastric ulcers were randomly given antacids only; eighteen were given antacids plus vitamin A 3 x 50,000 IU orally; and 22 were given antacids, vitamin A and cyproheptadine 3 x 4 mg orally daily. After four weeks, ulcers had completely healed in 3/16 (18%) in the antacid group; 7/18 (38%) in the vitamin A group; and 8/22 (36%) in the vitamin A plus cyproheptadine group. There was also an increase in size of remaining ulcers in group one but not in groups two and three. *Patty E et al. Controlled trial of vitamin A in gastric ulcer. Letter, Lancet 2:876, 1982.*

IF YOU HAVE AN ULCER, DON'T......

- Drink Regular Coffee
- Drink Decaffeinated Coffee
- Drink Tea
- Drink Alcohol
- Drink Milk
- Eat High Sugar Foods

All the above increase hydrochloric acid secretion! This aggravates ulcers.

Colitis

Colitis and its close relative **ulcerative colitis** can be a devastating experience. This condition usually begins with **diarrhea** combined with **pain** and **muscular spasms** in the bowel. As the disease progresses to ulceration, **blood** begins to show up in the stool.

Dehydration, malnutrition, loss of electrolyte balance and a host of other changes can take place in the body. **Depression** and **emotional instability** are characteristic of the condition, and there is a controversy as to whether the emotional symptoms are a causative factor or an effect of the disease.

The suffix "itis" means inflammation. In order to understand this disorder, we need to understand why one would have inflammation of the bowel.

Inflammation is usually a response to irritation. If we have an irritation in the colon, where did it come from?

Genetics of Colitis

In order to cloud up the issue greatly, let's look at the statistics and see who gets this kind of condition most frequently.

Caucasians suffer from colitis 3 times as often and Asians or Blacks

Jews suffer from colitis 4 times as often as Non-Jewish Caucasians

One could almost say that there must be something peculiar to the Jewish genetic pattern that predisposes one to the condition. Or does it mean that there is a ritual or belief in the Jewish religion that is involved? Such questions are not easily answered but can be compared to the fact that people on a primitive diet never get colitis. So is a dietary factor the most important predisposing element?

The most noticeable difference in the primitive diet and the diet of the Jew is sugar. Among all the civilized nations, Israel consumes more sugar per capita than any – an astounding **140 pounds of sucrose per person per year**. Considering children, diabetics and health food-conscious individuals, this would mean that some are consuming an astonishing three-quarters of a pound of sugar per day.

The significance of this is best summed up by an article in *Lancet*, one of the premier medical journals: *"A diet high in refined carbohydrate is implicated in the etiology of ulcerative colitis and certain other diseases of the colon. It is suggested that spasm of the smooth muscle is the common pathogenetic mechanism, and the strength of the spasm producing increased pressure in the colonic lumen or wall and the length of time for which the colon has been affected are believed to determine the type of disease resulting. A diet high in refined carbohydrate allows the intense muscle spasm to occur because the physical buffering effect of fecal bulk is considerably reduced."*

Lactose Intolerance Factor

There is a condition which afflicts approximately 5 to 10% of the population which involves an intolerance to the sugar found in milk, namely **lactose**. If the intestinal tract does not contain an enzyme known as **lactase**, the presence of milk sugar will produce gas, spasms of the bowel and often diarrhea. Obviously many of these symptoms are similar to that of colitis. This condition is called **"lactose intolerance"** and is treated with the addition of the enzyme lactase or the avoidance of milk and milk-containing foods.

Lactose intolerance was found in 25-35% of patients with inflammatory bowel disease which is a five times increase over average. Thus it would seem that if you have colitis in any of its forms, you might check to see if your symptoms are worse after drinking milk or eating milk-containing foods.

If that is true you should consider using lactase tablets with every meal that contains milk or just avoid milk altogether. *(Note: Such lactose intolerance does not include butter but may include cheeses.)*

It should be more and more clear that colitis is a condition that easily leads to more serious complications such as ulcerative colitis. Anything that benefits one will also benefit the other.

Vitamin E and Colitis

The following bit of research indicates the potential benefit supplementation of specific nutrients can have on disease conditions.

Three patients with nonspecific ulcerative colitis failed to respond to a twelve week combined treatment program consisting of a low carbohydrate, moderately high protein and fat diet, removal of foods to which they may have been sensitive, nutritional supplementation, stress reduction and spinal manipulation.

All therapeutic measures except for the low carbohydrate, moderately high protein and fat diet, wheat germ 4-6 tbls./day and yeast 1 tbls./day were discontinued, and alpha tocopherol pearls 40 IU/kg/day were added to the treatment program. Within 2 weeks all 3 patients experienced a rapid decrease in the amount of blood lost per bowel action, and 2/3 patients reported a substantial and rapid decrease in the amount of mucous present with each evacuation. The distressing, constant urge to evacuate was almost gone within four weeks.

All reported a marked lessening in the number of daily bowel movements and non-formed stools. Proctosigmoid examinations revealed less weeping of blood and less swelling in the rectal and sigmoid mucosa with a decrease in both the area and in the amount of capillary seepage. After 8 weeks, 2/3 patients had no rectal capillary oozing, excessive mucous production or inflammation.

One patient showed a small amount of capillary bleeding but the area of hemotumescent rectal mucous membrane showed continued shrinkage. By the 12th week all patients showed total healing of the rectal and sigmoid mucosa with no evidence of capillary bleeding or inflammation and bowel actions had returned to normal. *Hood RP Nonspecific ulcerative colitis: Successful treatment with d-alpha tocopherol. Digest of Chiropractic Economics Sept./Oct., 1984.*

What You Should Do If You Have A Colitis Disorder

1. Eat a high fiber diet.
2. Reduce the amount of sugar in your diet drastically.
3. Determine if milk or milk products affect your condition negatively – if so either eliminate them or add the enzyme lactase when you consume them.
4. Use 40 IU of vitamin E per kg of weight – 3000 IU if you weigh 150 lbs. – on a daily basis. Use 1000 IU per meal.
5. We have not discussed this but it is extremely important that the individual who suffers from colitis should make every effort to reduce any stress in their life. From a nutritional point of view, pantothenic acid, potassium, magnesium, calcium and vitamin C could be all important. A broad spectrum multi-vitamin/mineral product could supply all these factors.

Colitis and ulcerative colitis does not have to destroy your life as it has for so many others. Following the guidelines presented can alter the course of this disease and restore normal function.

Reduce sugar consumption
Increase vitamin E use
Check for lactose intolerance
Increase fiber in the diet
Reduce stress in your life
Use a broad spectrum
vitamin/mineral combination

Diverticulitis

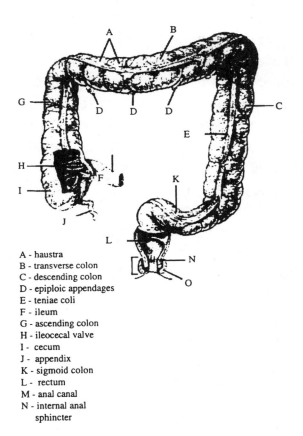

A - haustra
B - transverse colon
C - descending colon
D - epiploic appendages
E - teniae coli
F - ileum
G - ascending colon
H - ileocecal valve
I - cecum
J - appendix
K - sigmoid colon
L - rectum
M - anal canal
N - internal anal
    sphincter

The above represents the large intestine as we would like to have it in place in our body. Unfortunately the ideal is rarely seen in the human body – this large bowel is often looped and entangled, causing all kinds of problems. On the next page you will see a representation of how diverticula might appear on a cut segment of this tube.

Diverticula are small herniations or ruptures of the colon wall. The wall does not break but creates a small pouch similar to what a child might create by squeezing a balloon. **Diverticulosis** is the name of the disease when you have many diverticula.

Some patients with diverticulosis experience no symptoms but most complain of abdominal distention, cramping pain, diarrhea or constipation or one followed by the other. Those symptoms should be familiar – they kind of sound like colitis, don't they? That is why doctors need to take x-rays to differentiate between these two diseases.

If the little herniations become infected because fecal material is trapped and bacteria create an inflammation or infection, the condition is known as **diverticulitis**. If the condition gets this advanced you will have lots of symptoms!

Diverticula may occur anywhere along the small or large intestine but most frequently are found in the descending (sigmoid) portion of the colon. They are usually quite small but can reach one inch in diameter and no more than one to two inches in length. They are normally found in people over the age of forty and become much more common by the time you reach sixty years of age.

Here is a schematic representation of what a diverticula looks like:

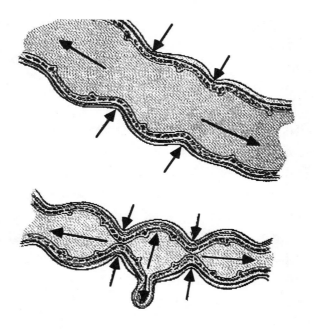

Mechanism by which low-fiber, low bulk diets
might generate diverticula is shown schematically.
Where colon contents are bulky (top) muscular
contractions exert pressure longitudinally. If
lumen is smaller (bottom), contractions can
produce occlusion and exert pressure against colon
wall, which may produce a diverticular "blowout."

Theory As To Cause

There is a very plausible theory proposed by some researchers that implicates a low fiber diet as being the major cause of diverticular disease. The theory proposes that the decreased stool size resulting from decreased fiber intake leads to increased intracolonic pressure which causes the wall of the colon to "pouch" and begins the process.

This theory flies in the face of the old opinion of most doctors which was based upon surgeon's observations. When diverticula perforated and required surgery, the surgeon would often find undigested fragments of fiber near the area and conclude that the fiber had aggravated the condition. When these observations were shared with the family care physician he agreed and began to caution his patients on not eating too much fiber because it "scratched or inflamed" the diverticula. Thus was born the "low roughage" diet for this condition.

As this opinion was reversed and some innovative doctors gave moderate to high fiber diet advice, several interesting changes were noted. Patients defecated easier, had less pain and less distention when the dietary fiber was increased. The swiftly passed soft stool subjected the colon to less strain and did not favor the development of more diverticula. It was found that the consumption of 1 heaping tablespoon of bran with each meal relieved the symptoms of the disease for most patients.

I know that for most of you this is the exact opposite of any advice you may have previously received. It is unfortunate that a majority of doctors still advise a "soft" diet, encouraging the use of relatively "foodless" refined flours, cooked, mushy foods rather than whole grains and raw fruits and vegetables.

PLEASE NOTE: There will often be an initial increase in intestinal gas from a change from bland, soft foods to a high fiber diet. This comes from a certain amount of fermentation in the lower tract because of the change in the content of the food you are eating and is very soon accommodated to and the gas disappears.

If you have wheat allergy and cannot use whole wheat or wheat bran, then use psyllium husk, oat bran or some other form of bulk. It is important that you understand that fiber is not digestible in the intestinal tract. Because of its makeup, fiber absorbs and holds water as it passes through the small intestine. This water content swells the fiber into several times its original volume. It is this swelling with water that makes the stool contents soft and easy to pass as well as helping to fill the colon so that the peristaltic contractions can easily move the material toward the rectum.

Diagnosis

There are two primary ways to make a positive diagnosis of diverticular disease:

1. X-Ray (preceded by a barium enema)
2. Endoscopy, in this instance sigmoidoscopy, a flexible fiber optic device which allows the doctor to see the interior of the colon.

Diverticula may become highly inflamed and become abscessed. This could leak and contaminate nearby pelvic organs such as the bladder or vagina, or a general peritonitis which could be fatal can develop. If such occurs the only avenue is surgery.

Diverticular Summary

It should be very apparent that the condition of diverticulitis, or any of its variations, is not something you want to allow to take its own course. There are just a few rules to follow and the condition can easily be remanded to an "onlooker" status.

Avoid Alcohol
Eat a Diet High in Fiber
Add Bran or Psyllium Husk Up to
Three Tablespoonfuls Daily

Constipation

Constipation is following diverticular disease in sequence because the reason for constipation is the exact same reason as for diverticular disease. In my 35 years in counselling people with health problems, I am constantly amazed at the number of individuals who suffer from constipation.

Many of them have developed an addiction to laxatives or enemas in order to move their bowels. Telling them to stop the use of these non-recommended procedures results in potentially serious consequences, so here are the facts you ought to know about this very prevalent condition.

Constipation means different things to different individuals. However, a good definition would be: **"Constipation is a lack of easy defecation on a regular daily basis when a reasonable amount of food is consumed."**

All too often doctors and other health advisors casually shrug off this condition, saying that it is totally normal for some people to only have two or three bowel movements per week. I hold that this is not only incorrect advice but potentially dangerous advice. Food normally moves through the digestive tract in 20 hours more or less. Thus, you should have a bowel movement 20 hours after any meal of significance.

The problem some individuals have is that the meals they eat are so low in fiber content that there is very little bulk reaching the large intestine and what there is does not contain enough moisture. So hard, small pieces are formed which do not move.

Another contributory factor is lack of exercise. A daily exercise program has been successful for many who have suffered from chronic constipation for years. I do not believe that exercise without fiber can be of any great value, but the exercise will certainly cause the person to drink more water and that is a very good result as it pertains to constipation.

An overlooked cause is certain medications that the individual may have been using. This is usually noticeable since the constipation and the beginning of the medicine are coincidental. The medicines which produce a paralyzing effect on the muscles of the colon include any of the morphine or codeine compounds, the mineral iron, aluminum and even calcium. So the use of aluminum and calcium containing antacids could be a cause of slow bowels.

I should not overlook the possibility of a blockage in the intestinal tract as a cause of constipation. This will usually come on suddenly and be accompanied by bloating and discomfort. It could signify something as serious as cancer or it may just be an accumulation of hardened feces that have become literally locked in position and will not allow other contents to move through.

Certain neuromuscular diseases can also lead to constipation because the nerve signal doesn't get to the muscles to move the contents of the gut along.

Multiple sclerosis, Parkinson's Disease and trauma to the spinal cord causing lower limb paralysis are some of the more common examples.

A history of constipation also is a factor, in that the walls of the colon will expand and require more bulk to activate the peristaltic action of the bowel wall. Constipation is all too casually viewed by the average person. It can contribute to **headaches**, a general feeling of **lassitude** and without a doubt it contributes to the **toxic load** in the blood stream as more and more compounds are absorbed through the wall of the colon. Women who are constipated have a **five-fold increase in breast cancer**. Such statistics should be reason enough to change your diet to one which does not predispose to slow passage time through the colon.

Laxatives

Laxatives are common remedies for constipation. Laxative foods such as prunes are an acceptable practice but one should be well aware that **all laxatives are irritating** and their action comes from the degree of irritation they produce in the colon. Because laxative foods are not just concentrated irritants and are diluted with many other factors which are beneficial (such as fiber) they may be used without concern. The "small but mighty" laxative pills are **concentrated irritants** that can create not only a dependence but also a need for ever increasing amounts.

My advice is to avoid laxatives except where absolutely necessary.

Enemas

An enema is the introduction into the rectal area of a solution which will produce evacuation of the contents of the colon. Historically they have consisted of solutions of soap, epsom salt or other ingredients which will produce the desired action.

The occasional or even regular use of enemas is welcome and can be very beneficial for the patient who cannot exercise and who is incapacitated for reasons of illness. There has recently been a surge of interest in the use of various preparations as an enema for reasons of detoxification.

I have no quarrel with the one time use of this in the individual who has a regular bowel movement, but remember that most of the ingredients of such enemas are also irritating to the colon - that's why they work so well in producing an evacuation.

It should also be perfectly clear that enemas usually work only on the lower end of the colon and will not unblock a problem that resides in the beginning portions of the colon. Such problems should be dealt with by using a very high liquid, high fiber approach to soften the contents so they may move along.

Rectal Suppositories

Rectal suppositories are a godsend on trips when the family often gets constipated. Change of diet, inactivity and less fluid consumed create the problem. The use of enemas may not be convenient, but inserting one or two glycerine suppositories can be easy and effective. They come in both adult and children sizes and are not something you want to use in place of the good habits listed below, but are certainly an option when needed.

Summary

Constipation is a prevalent problem that is a factor in many other conditions. It should be easy to correct in most circumstances by following these simple steps:

1. **Always eat a high fiber diet containing 4 cups of vegetables and 1 cup of fruit daily; also eat a bowl of whole grain cereal every morning.**
2. **Exercise by walking 30 minutes every day.**
3. **Consume a minimum of 2 quarts (liters) of water every day.**
4. **Use wheat bran, oat bran, psyllium husk powder or other high fiber bran if you have a history of constipation. Up to 20 or more grams can be used in a single day provided <u>enough water is consumed.</u>**

HEMORRHOIDS

Hemorrhoids, commonly known as *piles*, are varicose veins of the anal area. They are similar to the twisted and swollen veins visible on some people's legs, especially in older women who have had several children. When these varicosities occur before the anal sphincter they are called **internal hemorrhoids**. Usually these are asymptomatic with the exception that they may sometimes bleed. You can usually tell hemorrhoidal blood in the stool by its bright red color. Blood from further up the colon will usually be darker.

External hemorrhoids are after the anal sphincter and protrude outside. They can often become so engorged with blood that the individual cannot sit down because of the pain. Even lying down may be uncomfortable. The only relief comes when the hemorrhoid(s) burst open, releasing the blood and pressure.

Many annoying symptoms are associated with external hemorrhoids, including **burning and itching.** If they are prevalent, they interfere with proper hygiene and washing after a stool is recommended.

HEMORRHOIDS

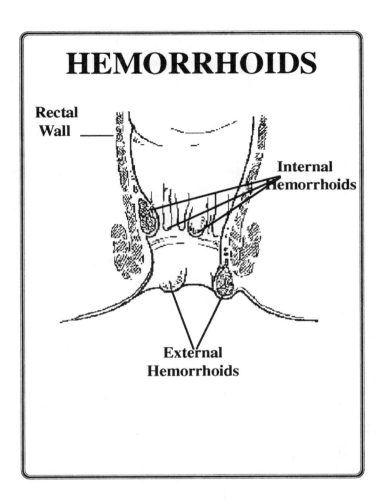

Rectal Wall

Internal Hemorrhoids

External Hemorrhoids

INSIDE VIEW OF RECTUM
AND ANUS

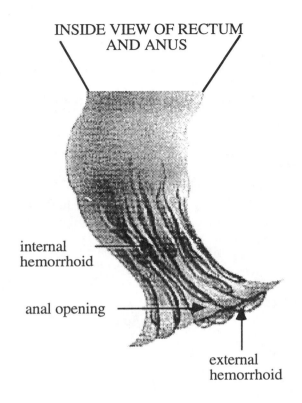

internal
hemorrhoid

anal opening

external
hemorrhoid

As mentioned, it is the external hemorrhoids which are the most painful and aggravating. The depiction above is not really as bad as many external hemorrhoids I have seen in some thirty-five years. Many of the protrusions are over one inch in length and regularly engorge themselves with blood whenever the individual strains at stool.

They also require washing the area after every bowel movement or the material which will adhere after wiping with dry toilet paper sets up an irritation that is unbearable.

Causes

The most frequent cause is straining during bowel movements, which is most common among people who are constipated or pregnant. People with liver disease such as cirrhosis may also develop hemorrhoids due to increased pressure in the veins of the intestine.

Many people believe that hemorrhoids can be caused by working in a sedentary occupation, sitting on hard, cold surfaces, standing for prolonged periods, or suffering from diarrhea. These factors are **not responsible** for hemorrhoids but will seriously aggravate a hemorrhoid that has **thrombosed** (swollen with blood) until it bursts.

Creams and Ointments

There are many different types of creams and ointments which are sold to relieve hemorrhoids. Some contain cortisone *(an anti-inflammatory)*, others contain xylocaine *(an anesthetic)* and still others claim that they will shrink the hemorrhoid tag. *(Some years ago a fad developed which consisted of ladies applying a popular hemorrhoidal remedy to their faces on the belief that if it would shrink hemorrhoids then it would also shrink their wrinkles. I don't believe it worked but it was not harmful.)* I am also not totally convinced *(not having heard of actual shrinking taking place)* that these creams shrink hemorrhoids.

But they all do provide a modicum of relief and should not be condemned.

Forms of Surgery

Regular surgical removal, **hemorrhoidectomy,** of external hemorrhoids is not as common as it used to be. It can be done with a scalpel or with a laser. A procedure called **ligation**, a tying off of the hemorrhoid with a rubber band to strangulate it, is becoming more common. **Cryosurgery** uses liquid nitrogen or carbon dioxide to freeze the hemorrhoid and thus destroy the tissue.

Hot Sitz Baths

The time honored remedy for hemorrhoids is heat, usually in the form of a hot tub. This does work and provides temporary relief. I must share the most dramatic and effective relief that I have seen in my entire practice and observational career.

An inventor who suffered from hemorrhoids himself and who recognized that heat was doing some good for him, thought that he could devise a better way of heating the area which was giving him trouble. After all, it was really difficult to get the water right on the affected area and maintain the temperature which was necessary to get relief.

He devised a stainless steel probe which could be inserted from two to three inches into the anal opening which was connected to a rechargeable battery. *(He correctly surmised that it was not the best idea to be plugged into an electrical socket in case of a current surge.)* The probe is capable of achieving temperatures of 112 degrees Fahrenheit which is very comfortable in that area. *(Temperatures of 130 degrees fahrenheit are tolerated quite well.)*

The use of this for one hour per day, or for two sessions the first one or two days is probably the best thing that ever happened to an external hemorrhoid sufferer. I have given this unit to patients for temporary use and they are willing to pay any price just to keep it. One of the real miracles for this condition!

Hemorrhoid Summary

If you have hemorrhoids do the following:

1. **Do everything I suggested for constipation, because if you are not constipated you will not have engorged hemorrhoids.**

2. **Find a doctor who knows of the device I spoke about *(or one who will call me for the information)* and get a few treatments or purchase one for yourself. *(Tip: I am now using this unit successfully for benign prostatic hypertrophy with great success. It's much preferable to an operation and is really quite inexpensive.)***

HIATAL HERNIA

Hiatal hernia is an outpouching of a portion of the stomach into the chest through the esophageal opening in the diaphragm. The illustrations which follow show the different types of hiatal hernia possibilities.

Hiatal Hernia

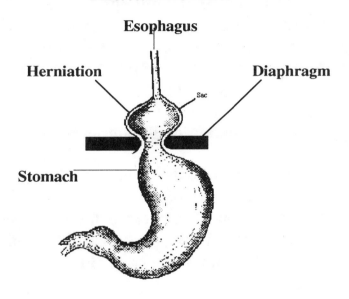

This hernia is called a **sliding hiatal hernia** in which part of the stomach pushes up around the esophagus and herniates through the diaphragm into the thorax.

HIATAL HERNIA

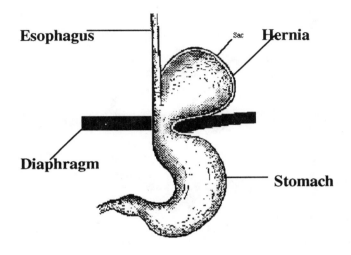

Esophagus

Sac Hernia

Diaphragm

Stomach

This herniation is called a **paraesophageal** or "next to the esophagus" hernia. It is a protrusion of the stomach through a torn esophageal opening into the thorax.

HIATAL HERNIA

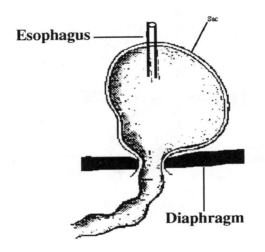

Esophagus

Sac

Diaphragm

This is a depiction of the worst hiatal hernia called a gastroesophageal hernia in which the lower esophagus and part of the stomach protrude through the diaphragm into the thorax.

Symptoms of Hiatal Hernia

Most of the symptoms of hiatal hernia occur approximately 2 hours after a full meal. It is made much worse if the sufferer is in a reclining position. What literally occurs is that the weakened portion of the diaphragm allows a part of the stomach to escape into the thorax when the pressure in the stomach is too high.

This high stomach pressure comes from fermentation from improper combining of foods, from achlorhydria *(lack of hydrochloric acid)*, or just from eating too much.

Remember that the diaphragm is the strongest muscle in the body. As part of the stomach slides past a tear in this muscle and pouches outward, imagine the pressure this muscle can put on the pouch. You will have continual pain from the strangling of the pouch until the pouch drains backward and relaxes into its normal position.

Another cause of pain will be the acid stomach contents pushing upward into the esophagus which is not protected against such acidity by heavy mucous membranes.

This pain will often be so intense and will so mimic a heart attack that patients often admit themselves into a hospital convinced that they are experiencing a heart attack.

Hiatal Hernia Suggestions

1. Use digestive enzymes with every meal.
2. Eat smaller meals, more often if necessary.
3. Do not go to bed within three hours of a heavy meal. If you must lie down, prop your upper body at a 45 degree angle.

You will never cure a hiatal hernia, but following the suggestions above should make the condition livable. Surgery can be performed in some instances and is advisable if the circumstances are severe.

GALL STONES and CHOLECYSTITIS

Cholecystitis is an inflammation of the gall bladder usually produced by gall stones. The gall bladder is a sac located under the liver which collects bile for release when a fatty meal is eaten. The bile is used to emulsify the fat particles so they are smaller and easier for the enzyme lipase to break them down.

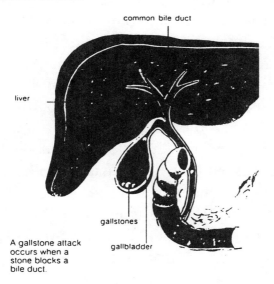

common bile duct

liver

gallstones

gallbladder

A gallstone attack occurs when a stone blocks a bile duct.

Why gall stones form in the gallbladder is not really known, but it is known that the major ingredient in most gall stones is cholesterol. Before you panic and blame cholesterol, please be aware that the elimination or reduction of cholesterol in the diet does not prevent or even reduce the formation of gall stones in those who are prone to form them.

So what does cause the stone to form? One can theorize that it is probably the concentration of the bile that produces the stone. Stagnation of bile in the gall bladder in a viscosity too thick to readily flow down the tube to the small intestine could be the cause. If that theory is correct then we must determine what "thins" the bile.

A nutrient called choline, has the ability to do just that - liquefy the bile so that it flows more freely. It is an essential component of lecithin and also of acetylcholine, a neurotransmitter. In order to thin the bile adequately, supplemental amounts close to 3 grams daily must be used of this nutrient.

In any single day the liver may produce as much as three cups (700 milliliters) of bile. In those who form gall stones, the cholesterol component of bile seems to fall out of solution and crystallize into the stones. This propensity to form crystals is probably due to a missing or deficient ingredient which I theorize to be choline. Choline probably holds cholesterol in solution in the bile just as magnesium holds calcium in solution in the blood stream.

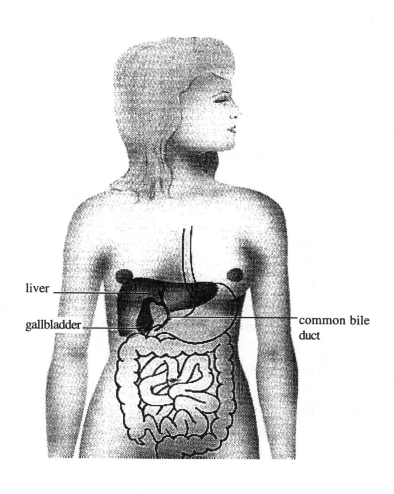

liver

gallbladder

common bile duct

Symptoms of Gall Stones

One of the most intense pains known to man is the passing of either a gall stone or a kidney stone. But long before this happens the stone bearer will have noticed a severe, steady pain in the upper abdomen. It will often last about 20 minutes but can last up to four hours. There may be pain between the shoulder blades or in the right shoulder. There may be nausea and/or vomiting. Some will perspire heavily and become violently ill.

All in all, gall bladder stones or stones in the bile duct are not fun and can cause tremendous discomfort.

Suggestions for Gall Stones

1. **Use <u>3 grams of choline</u> on a daily basis for several months, then reduce the dosage.**
2. **Find a doctor who will prescribe <u>chenodeoxycholic acid</u> to help you dissolve the stones you have.**
3. **Restrict the amount of fats in your diet and use a digestive aid containing bile salts with every meal.**

PARASITES

In past years the incidence of intestinal parasites was quite high, but in today's society the very thought that one might have parasites causes a shudder. Unfortunately **you** probably **have parasites**. It may not be nice to think about but here are the facts:

1. If you had a microscope and could look at just a small part of your external skin, you would see all kinds of creatures busy living off you. There are mites, lice and fungi which inhabit your skin.

2. Internally we need to concern ourselves with tapeworms, flukes, roundworms, pinworms, hookworms, internal viruses, fungi, bacteria and protozoa. No one is immune.

The concentration of these creatures which use your blood or other body parts to maintain their life is a critical factor. Under normal circumstances your body's defense system will keep their population down and you can live with them in relative comfort. But allow them to multiply explosively and you will be sick!

It is estimated that 80 percent of all children are infected with pinworms. These one-fourth inch long pests are the major cause of stomach aches in children. They live in the large intestine and the female comes out at night to lay eggs outside the anus. The resultant itch makes the child scratch. This contact allows the eggs to be picked up under the fingernails and reinfest the child or those who they play with. This can come about through direct or indirect contact - such as shared toys.

Pinworm Diagnosis

Since the female comes out at night to lay her eggs, you can inspect your child's anal area about one or two hours after they have gone to sleep. The small white worm is often easily visible. You can also see the worms in the stool sometimes or you can take a stool sample and send it in to a laboratory or you can take a piece of scotch tape and wipe the anal area, fold it and send it to the lab for the presence of the eggs.

A pretty positive diagnosis can be attained by just observing a child who often complains of abdominal pain, who is restless at night or who grinds their teeth during sleep. Doctors can give you a relatively harmless vermifuge, or you might want to try garlic and/or black walnut shell capsules.

I really want to emphasize that an incredible percentage of individuals have some form of intestinal parasites. It is just good common sense to give yourself an herbal vermifuge treatment every year. This is particularly important for children and can make a big difference in their disposition and state of health.